Yoga for All

See how this simple art form of exercise can improve your health and strengthen your body.

Copyright
Lewis Stout

Table of Contents

Introduction

We need to place more emphasis on health and disease treatment. Many drugs only treat the symptoms of the disease, not the underlying cause. The causes of many chronic diseases are still under research.

Yoga therapy can help us here. Yoga focuses on treating the root cause of disease. It works slowly, delicately, and wonderfully.

Chapter 1:
Basics of Yoga

Overview

Yoga means "union" in Sanskrit, the ancient Indian language where yoga originated. We can think of it as a union of body, mind, and soul. Yoga is the practice of postures and postures.

Basic Information
Many people think that yoga is just a stretching exercise. While these are certainly stretching exercises, yoga is actually about balancing the body by developing both strength and flexibility.

While yoga classes at gyms usually focus on the purely physical benefits of yoga, yoga classes at yoga centers focus on the spiritual aspects. Some people find that the physical practice of yoga can be a gateway to a journey of spiritual discovery, while others simply enjoy a great low-impact workout that makes them feel great. Whatever your temperament, you can find a yoga class that suits your style.

Yoga has many benefits and is a great way to increase flexibility, build muscle strength, and deal with tension. Stretching your body in new ways increases your body's flexibility and increases the mobility of your muscles and joints. Yoga poses require you to support your weight in new ways to improve both strength and muscle tone.

Physical activity is great for relieving tension, and this is especially true for yoga. Because it requires concentration, everyday problems, big and small, seem to disappear by themselves while practicing yoga.

Yoga is divided into eight sections known as the eight "limbs" of yoga. Each link is connected to an aspect of a healthy and fulfilling life, and each link builds on the one before it. You may be surprised to hear that only one limb affects the performance of a yoga pose.

Chapter 2:
What is Hot Yoga?

Summary

As the title suggests, this form of yoga is primarily practiced in hot, humid environments with a constant temperature.

Behind the Heat

Other effects can occur when this particular feature is incorporated into a yoga session. Interestingly, although yoga is a very gentle and slow art form, some people may end up feeling refreshed and even a little sweaty after a session.

Practicing a style of hot yoga is also about actually sweating out unnecessary negative elements in your body. None of those who use this style consider excessive sweating to be an unpleasant side effect, in fact, most welcome it.

Hot yoga is a series of yoga poses specifically designed to be performed in a hot or heated room. The temperature of the environment where hot yoga is performed is often kept at around 95 to 100 degrees.

It is said that the temperature alone causes a lot of sweating, and when combined with yoga exercises, the body can absorb and release different levels of heat, resulting in an individual's body becoming more supple and supple. I am.

**Here are some of the benefits
you can get from a hot yoga style.**

• Increases the mobility of joints,
muscles, ligaments, and other
supporting structures of the body.
· When the environment is warmed,
capillaries dilate more easily, so
tissues and muscles are more
effectively supplied with oxygen.

• Increased sweating improves
peripheral blood circulation.

• Metabolism accelerates

• The cardiovascular system is kept at
a comfortable level but trained more
intensely

• Sweating increases detoxification
and removes toxins from the
skin.Chapter 3:
How Yoga Can Help Stress Disorders
and Hyperactivity Disorders

Overview

Yoga is an increasingly popular form of exercise around the world. Yoga is gaining in popularity because it can be done in a small space does not require a gym membership, and is likely to continue to grow.

In addition to the practical benefits that yoga provides, regular participation also benefits your body and mind. Yoga combines exercise and meditation, making it a versatile approach to gaining control over multiple areas of need.

Calm

Yoga is another way to help people with hyperactivity problems. This art form teaches individuals to increase their concentration and promotes mental and physical discipline, thus creating an element of increased confidence and focus.

Balance is a common technique in yoga exercises. Many poses involve shifting your weight to different parts of your body and maintaining balance while breathing deeply. Breathing control exercises are associated with coping with emotions and help restore oxygen to the brain.

All of this further trains the individual to slow down and focus. In hyperactive states, the mind-body connection is impaired, so yoga always promotes self-awareness and control while making the mind more disciplined.

Yoga reduces stress, which is another factor for people who already suffer from hyperactivity. Yoga improves an individual's ability to synchronize the overactive nervous system and eliminate stimulation.

Another benefit of practicing yoga regularly is increasing your strength and building stronger, leaner muscles. Strength-building exercises also promote sleep and help regulate unhealthy sleep habits. When you don't get enough sleep, your brain's problem-solving processes slow down. This is another way yoga helps the mind function at a higher level. Yoga promotes concentration and creativity, ensuring good health and peace of mind.

Chapter 4:
Relieve Arthritis Symptoms with Yoga

Summary

Dealing with arthritis can be very stressful and painful. Most arthritis patients eagerly seek medical or alternative treatments to address their potentially debilitating illness.

Pain Relief

In most cases, a combination of a proper exercise program and other necessary prescription supplements is recommended. Those who dared to start practicing yoga found that they were able to achieve excellent recovery rates from this disease of arthritis.

Over time, yoga has developed into a popular method for treating arthritis. Yoga provides a gentle exercise routine for arthritis patients who already suffer from constant pain.

Each movement in yoga has a corresponding counter-movement, which helps target the different muscles and joints affected by arthritis. Many people who have tried yoga see almost immediate pain relief after just a few supervised sessions.

With the help of yoga, you can address deep-seated resentments by focusing on restoring balance to your chakra system.

When yoga is used as a treatment for arthritis, the genes in your body that protect you from pain and discomfort can work more efficiently, creating a relaxing effect. This provides patients with immediate relief from pain caused by arthritis.

Some researchers associate arthritis with the development of deep-seated resentment within an individual. This chakra system is therefore a major energy vortex located along the spine and is associated with energies of compassion and love towards self and others.

Yoga helps to give the body a chance to rid itself of this negative energy pattern that causes arthritis at the deepest level.

Chapter 5:
Yoga Helps Relieve Back Pain

Summary

People often turn to painkillers and other medically prescribed treatments to control or reduce back pain. All these foreign substances can be avoided if an individual decides to try the art form of yoga to treat back pain. Yoga is natural and has no side effects from prescription drugs.

Relief

When used correctly, yoga can effectively cure lower back pain by stretching and training muscles and joints. All you need is a few small yoga exercises every day.
Once you have narrowed down the position that is best for lower back pain treatment, you can practice the movements at any time.

To solve back problems, you need to look at certain factors. Incorrect posture, incorrect movements, poor body mechanics, repetitive and intense movements of joints and muscles, disc injuries, ligament injuries, and inflammation are just some of these problems.

A properly monitored combination of yoga movements can correct all of the above, some gradually and some more quickly. Through various yoga poses, you can target and realign specific

muscle and joint areas to restore your body's center position.
The most common yoga poses for treating lower back pain include the locust pose, cobra pose, and some poses of the tadasana regiment.

In addition to various yoga exercises to strengthen your back muscles and strengthen your posture, we also recommend incorporating other regular exercises into your daily life. Simple exercises such as swimming and light strength training are good ways to build and strengthen your back area.

As we get older, we also need to be careful about the strain placed on our lower back when lifting heavy objects or doing strenuous exercise or work.

Chapter 6:
Spiritual Healing through Yoga

Summary

Everything in life is the contribution of her two elements: cause and effect. Using drugs to treat symptoms or illnesses only addresses the effects of the problem, not the root cause.

This will cause the problem to recur and require further treatment. This is a vicious cycle, and most people take it for granted because drugs often work quickly and satisfactorily to solve the problem.

Your Mind

Most of the root causes of illness, disease, and discomfort are due to improper diet, chemicals taken in the form of medicines, or the general attitude of the individual. Yoga techniques address these very important aspects through postures, poses, and deep breathing exercises.

In addition to yoga exercise therapy, other aspects of yoga can be specially trained. This is the spiritual aspect of yoga. Spiritual Yoga teaches us to adopt a simple attitude toward life and not to be preoccupied with constantly striving for material things to achieve satisfaction.

Yoga teaches you how to connect with your inner person. Through poses and meditation, you can center your inner self and create a very powerful energy source that can provide the healing power needed to heal. Being able to tap into this inner strength should be the goal of spiritual harmony for everyone.

In the spiritual healing process, he works on three levels. The focus is on balancing the energies of the entire being and maintaining balance in consciousness. Using yoga for spiritual healing also has a positive impact on the overall interests of the individual in terms of reaction to external elements. Due to the peaceful and holistic nature that the person now has, it will hardly have any negative impact on his life.

Chapter 7:
Emotional Healing with Yoga

Summary

A person's emotional well-being is critical to maintaining good health and a good outlook on life. If a person's mental health is not at an optimal positive level, over time all other parts of the body begin to break down. This negative process is so subtle that few, if any, people are aware of the relationship.

Free your mind

All emotions are considered sacred. The problem lies in how we deal with these emotions. Through the practice of yoga, one learns to calm the body and mind, teaching the mind to achieve a level of peace and contentment. When this is well understood and learned, the process of emotional healing can occur.

A person with the emotional strength that comes from learning yoga learns the difference between reacting to a situation or conflict and reacting to it.

Emotional healing helps individuals develop the mindset that they can control their instinctive reactions to negative situations, such as anger, frustration, and sadness, and change them to more positive reactions to the situation. Helpful.

This allows yoga techniques to promote emotional healing from within and prevent negative energy from entering from the outside. In this way, the individual stays connected to the spirit and truth of his or her inner self.

Emotional healing through yoga means that the person no longer perceives the situation as a victim; rather, this ability gives the individual the strength to confidently strengthen their self-identity. Masu.

At the cellular level, even the cells of our body imprint corresponding emotions into our thoughts and reproduce them in our cellular structures. Therefore, linking your healing pattern to your current optimal level of healing brings out the positive elements in both your body and mind.

Chapter 8:
How to Practice Yoga Breathing

Summary

Breathing is the basis of life, and without it death is inevitable. You need to learn how to breathe properly as it is one of the most important parts of your life.

Yoga promotes this proper breathing. This is as important as science in oxygenating the blood and brain. These breathing techniques provide the ultimate in cleansing and self-discipline, encompassing both mind and body.

Proper Breathing

The main purpose of yoga breathing techniques is to prepare you physically and mentally for the meditative phase. In general, most people do not know how important it is to breathe correctly. Most people breathe very shallowly, which does not provide enough oxygen throughout the body, leading to various illnesses. Yoga breathing is the art of inhaling deeply until it almost fills your lungs, then exhaling slowly while focusing on the process.

Here are some simple steps for yoga breathing techniques.

• Choose a quiet, dimly lit location or a location with natural light.
• Use a comfortable yoga mat.
• Sit on your mat with your legs crossed and pulled toward your chest.
• Keep your back straight and your arms in a relaxed and comfortable position on your thighs.
• Touch your thumb and index finger with your palm facing down.
• Breathe deeply and focus on your breathing.
•Concentrate on breathing through your stomach area, not just your chest. We will focus on ensuring this.

• Once you reach the level, switch between cheat breathing and abdominal breathing.

•Place your index and middle fingers on your thumb with your ring and little fingers sticking out, press one nostril, inhale deeply, and exhale. Do this alternately with the other nostril.

Chapter 9:
Yoga Poses and Their Purpose

Summary

Each of the yoga poses represents different aspects that need to be considered in healing and improving an individual's overall health. Masu. Strengthening all parts of the body, including the abdominal muscles, and areas around and near the spinal cord, ensures better health.

Each pose in yoga teaches the body to support its weight, rather than relying on other muscles to share or shoulder the weight. It also helps strengthen your inner strength and self-confidence.

Pose

The mountain pose is one of the simplest and most used poses. Although it is said to be so simple that you can learn it directly from the book, this is not the recommended way to start yoga.
This posture is a good means of self-healing and relaxation.

Bird of Paradise poses strengthen your leg muscles. It also improves your balance by focusing on the muscles you need and not relying on other muscles. It also helps improve balance while relaxing the groin and hamstring muscles.

Bridge pose takes some getting used to, but it does wonders for your spine. In addition to its main purpose of strengthening the spine, it opens the rib cage, improves spinal flexibility, and stimulates the thyroid.

The cobra pose is a pose that focuses on the spine. It increases the flexibility of the spine and is effective in relieving lower back pain.

Dolphin Pose is similar to Dog Pose and is used to improve blood circulation. This is especially useful for people with wrist problems, which are common among pianists, computer users, and writers.

Dragonfly Pose, also known as Hummingbird Pose, is very difficult and requires a lot of practice, but once achieved, it helps strengthen arm and arm balance skills.

There are many other poses and the possibilities are endless if you want to explore further. However, to be effective, it is recommended to select and use only a few poses at a time.

Chapter 10:
Possible Side Effects of Yoga

Overview

As with most things, side effects are bound to occur if you do not take the time to understand the work being done. The same goes for yoga, which is known for its grace and gentleness, but it should be taken for granted and you should deviate from it until you understand the possible consequences of deviating from it.

What you need to know

Some yoga movements may seem simple at first glance, but they are made up of very difficult maneuvers. Therefore, it is very important to start your yoga adventure under the supervision of an experienced yoga practitioner.

If performed incorrectly, these poses can cause serious injury or simply be useless for what the individual is trying to accomplish.

We also recommend that you consult your doctor before considering participating in a yoga program. Some people do this without the critical advice of a doctor and mistakenly decide not to continue their ongoing treatment or medication and replace it with yoga. This exclusion is recommended and possible only if a positive result is obtained.

In addition to wrist, neck, and back pain, some people suffer from ligament tears and tendon and muscle injuries. Although it is rare, the side effects of dizziness may be described.

In some cases, stomach problems occur at the beginning of a series of yoga classes. One possible explanation for this stomach discomfort is that the discomfort is caused by not performing the prescribed poses in the correct order. There are also cases of nausea, stomach acid, and vomiting.

If you take your yoga practice too seriously and warning signs of discomfort are ignored and untreated, surprisingly serious consequences can occur, including internal bleeding, severe strains, and broken bones. In such cases, you should immediately seek medical attention.

Summary

Just discussing these topics can help reduce mental tension and change your mental attitude. Simple asanas help stretch and relax the entire body and neutralize tension.

Practicing yoga poses seriously is useful for all levels of experience.

From restoring balance, flexibility, equilibrium, health, and well-being in the body to cultivating mental calm, emotional balance, and inner strength.

On a physical level, yoga poses activate glands, organs, muscles, and nerves in ways that traditional exercise cannot.